Stretching Exercises for Seniors Over 60

50 Easy Stretches to Decrease Back pains and Reduce risk of Injury

<u>BONUS CHAPTER</u>

5 Minute Stretching Routines for Different Times of the Day

Nathan Anderson

Disclaimer

The information in the book is based on personal research and experience. The author advises readers to consult with their healthcare provider before making any dietary changes

For more information or to contact the author, please email:

fitstrideanderson@gmail.com

Table of Contents

CHAPTER 8: INCORPORATING STRETCHING INTO DAILY LIFE 81

Introduction

In the golden years of life, as our bodies' age, they often become more susceptible to the relentless grip of time. As the joints creak and the muscles ache, it is all too easy to succumb to a sedentary lifestyle, resigned to accepting a diminished state of well-being. But what if I told you that there is a way to unlock vitality, ease those persistent body pains, and regain a newfound sense of freedom? This is where the power of stretching comes into play.

Allow me to share with you the true life story of my Aunt Mary. My dear aunt Mary, is a vibrant woman who embodies the very essence of resilience, love, and joy. As the years crept up on her, she too found herself grappling with the relentless march of time. Back pains and nagging discomfort had become an all too familiar companion in her daily life, casting a shadow over the activities she once cherished.

However, Aunt Mary, like countless others yearning for relief, refused to surrender to the notion that aging meant surrendering her vitality. Together, we embarked on a journey to unlock the secrets to rejuvenate and reclaim her zest for life. During this eye-opening journey, we discovered the unexpected, yet transformative power of stretching.

Aunt Mary began incorporating gentle stretches into her daily activities, a deliberate and dedicated effort to address the needs of her aging body. At first, it was a mere act of faith for us. A flicker of hope amidst the shadows of pain and doubt. But as days turned into weeks, and weeks into months, an astonishing change began to unfold.

With each stretch, my aunt felt the tightness in her muscles gradually release, providing relief and liberation from the clutches of discomfort. A newfound suppleness started to infuse her being, reawakening her sense of physical freedom. Simple tasks that once seemed arduous became effortless once more. The once-forgotten joy of taking long walks basked in the familiar warmth of her heart. Not only did my Aunt Mary experience a reduction in back pains, she was no longer plagued by the fear of a fall or the unpredictable vulnerability that had cast its shadow over her days. The practice of stretching had become her armor against the perils of aging, fortifying her body, mind, and spirit.

My aunt's friends and companions began to notice the changes and soon, they too found solace in the power of stretching. Once resigned to languishing in the limitations of age, new life was breathed to them as they collectively embarked on a journey of self-care, vitality, and discovery.

Now, it is my privilege to share with you the wisdom, insights, and comprehensive stretching guide that emerged from Aunt Mary's extraordinary experience. Within the pages of this book, you will find a comprehensive collection of 50 easy stretches designed specifically for seniors over 60. These stretches have been handpicked to address the specific needs, challenges, and potential risks that come with aging, particularly focusing on reducing back pain and injury risks to the body.

So, my dear reader, whether you are a senior seeking relief or a caregiver looking to support your loved ones on their journey, I implore you to join us on this transformative exploration of the powers of stretching. Together, let us unlock the means to reclaim joy, vitality, and the extraordinary potential that lies within our aging bodies.

Chapter 1: Warm-Up Exercises before Stretching for Seniors

Before diving into the world of stretching, it is crucial for you to engage in a proper warm-up routine to prepare your body for the upcoming exercises. Here are some step-by-step explanations to ensure a safe and effective warm-up.

Routine 1: Joint Mobilization and Circulation

- **Step 1: March in Place**

To begin, stand tall with your feet hip-width apart.

Begin to march in place, lifting your feet off the

ground slightly and swinging your arms back and forth. Continue this movement for 1-2 minutes, gradually increasing the height of your knee lifts.

- **Step 2: Shoulder Rolls**

Stand upright with your feet shoulder-width apart. Gently roll your shoulders forward in a circular motion, completing 5 rotations. Then, reverse the direction and perform 5 shoulder rolls backward.

- **Step 3: Wrist and Ankle Circles**

Extend your arms out in front of you and gently rotate your wrists in a circular motion. Complete 5 rotations in one direction and then repeat in the opposite direction. Next, lift one foot off the ground and rotate your ankle in a circular motion. Complete 5 rotations before switching to the other foot.

- **Step 4: Neck Stretch**

Stand tall with your feet hip-width apart. Slowly tilt your head to the right, aiming to bring your right ear closer to your right shoulder. Hold this stretch for 10-15 seconds, then return to the starting position. Repeat on the left side.

Routine 2: Dynamic Movements

- **Step 1: Arm Circles**

Stand upright with your feet hip-width apart. Extend your arms out to the side with palms facing down. Begin to make small, controlled circles with your arms. Gradually increase the size of the circles. Reverse the direction of the circles after 10-15 seconds. Repeat for another 30 seconds.

- **Step 2: Leg Swings**

Stand beside a sturdy support (such as a chair or wall) and hold onto it for balance. Start by swinging your right leg forward and backward in a controlled motion. Perform 10 swings on each leg.

- **Step 3: Torso Twists**

Place your hands on your hips and stand with your feet shoulder-width apart. Slowly rotate your upper body to the right, allowing your hips and feet to follow naturally. Hold the twist for a moment before returning to the center. Repeat the twist to the left. Perform 10 twists on each side.

- **Step 4: Knee Lifts**

Stand tall with your feet hip-width apart. Lift your right knee toward your chest, aiming to bring it as close as possible to your chest. As you lower your lifted leg, immediately raise your left knee. Repeat this movement, alternating legs, for a total of 10 knee lifts on each side.

By incorporating these warm-up routines into your stretching practice, you ensure that your muscles and joints are adequately prepared for the exercises that follow. Remember to listen to your body and only perform movements that feel comfortable and within your range of motion. With a proper warm-up, you will enhance your overall stretching experience and minimize the risk of injuries.

Chapter 2: Upper Body Stretches

In this chapter, we will focus on stretching exercises specifically for the upper body. These stretches target the neck, shoulders, arms, and chest, aiming to improve flexibility, relieve muscle tension, and promote better posture. Whether you spend your days sitting at a desk or engaging in physical activities, these stretches will help relax and rejuvenate your upper body muscles. Remember to start with a gentle warm-up before proceeding with the stretches, as discussed earlier

Neck Stretches

1. Neck Tilt

Sit or stand upright with your spine in neutral alignment. Slowly tilt your head to the right, aiming to bring your right ear closer to your right shoulder. Avoid lifting the shoulder towards the ear. Hold this stretch for 15-20 seconds, feeling the gentle elongation on the opposite side of your neck. Return to the starting location and do the same on the other side.

2. Neck Rotation

Maintaining an upright posture, slowly rotate your head to the right, aiming to look over your shoulder.

Keep your shoulders stationary and avoid shrugging them. Hold this stretch for 15-20 seconds, feeling the stretch in the back of your neck. Return to the starting position and repeat the rotation to the left.

3. Chin to Chest

Sit or stand with good posture. Slowly lower your chin to your chest, feeling the stretch along the back of your neck. Avoid pressing down forcefully, as this stretch should be gentle. Hold for 15-20 seconds before slowly raising your head back to the starting position.

Shoulder Stretches

1. Shoulder Rolls

Place your feet shoulder-width apart and sit or stand tall. Begin by gently rolling your shoulders forward in a circular manner. Complete 5 rotations, then reverse the direction and perform 5 shoulder rolls backward. This exercise helps reduce tension in the shoulder muscles and increases flexibility.

2. Arm Across Chest

Extend your right arm straight in front of you, parallel to the ground. Keeping your arm straight, bring the right arm across your chest, using your left hand to gently guide it closer to your body. Hold this stretch for 15-20 seconds, feeling the stretch in your right shoulder and upper back. Repeat on the left side.

3. Shoulder Stretch with Arm Extension

Stand or sit up straight, your feet shoulder-width apart. Raise your right arm and bend it at the elbow, reaching your right hand toward the middle of your back. With your left hand, reach behind your back and try to clasp your right hand. If this is challenging, gently use a towel or strap to assist in the stretch. Hold for 15-20 seconds, feeling the stretch in your right shoulder and upper arm. Repeat on the left side.

Arm Stretches

1. Bicep Stretch

Stand tall with your feet shoulder-width apart. Extend your right arm straight in front of you, parallel to the ground, with the palm facing up. Bend your right elbow, bringing your forearm towards your body until you feel a gentle stretch in your bicep. Hold for 15-20 seconds before repeating on the opposite side.

2. Tricep Overhead Stretch

Stand or sit upright, grasping your right elbow with your left hand. Raise your right arm overhead, bending it at the elbow to reach towards your upper back. With your left hand, gently press your right elbow downwards, feeling the stretch in your tricep. Hold for 15-20 seconds before repeating on the opposite side.

3. Wrist Flexor Stretch

Extend your right arm straight in front of you, parallel to the ground, and flex your wrist, pointing your fingers towards the ground. Use your left hand to gently pull back on your right hand, feeling the stretch in the underside of your forearm. Hold for 15-20 seconds and switch to the left side.

Chest Stretches

1. Wall Chest Stretch

Stand facing a wall with your feet slightly wider than shoulder-width apart. Extend your right arm and place the palm of your hand against the wall. Slowly rotate your body away from the wall, feeling the stretch in the front of your chest and shoulder. Hold for 15-20 seconds before repeating on the opposite side.

2. Doorway Stretch

Stand in a doorway with your arms bent at 90-degree angles, placing your forearms and hands on the sides of the doorway. Step forward, allowing your chest to gently lean into the doorway. Feel the stretch across your chest and front shoulders. Hold for 15-20 seconds.

3. Pectoral Stretch

Place your feet shoulder-width apart and sit or stand tall. Clasp your hands behind your lower back, palms facing inward. Begin to lift your clasped hands away from your back, feeling the stretch in your chest and shoulders. Hold for 15-20 seconds, then release.

By incorporating these upper body stretches into your regular routine, you can improve flexibility, reduce muscle tension, and promote better posture. Remember to perform these exercises in a controlled manner, respecting your body's limitations. Enjoy the benefits that these stretches bring to your upper body health and well-being.

Chapter 3: Lower Body Stretches

Welcome to this chapter, where we will explore a series of lower body stretches to promote flexibility, improve muscular balance, and prevent injury. Our lower body plays a crucial role in daily activities, so it's incredibly important to keep these muscles and joints limber and healthy. In this chapter, we will target the hips, quadriceps, hamstrings, and calves, offering you a range of stretches to enhance your lower body mobility. Remember to perform a light warm-up before attempting these stretches, as discussed in earlier.

1. Seated Pigeon Pose

Start by sitting upright on the ground. Bend your right knee and cross your ankle over your left thigh, creating a figure-four shape. Flex your right foot to stabilize your ankle. Gently lean forward, keeping your back straight, until you feel a stretch in your right hip and gluteus area. Hold this stretch for 15-20 seconds and then repeat on the left side.

2. Butterfly Stretch

Sit on the ground so that the soles of your feet are touching. With your hands, grip your ankles or feet.

Gently press down on your thighs with your elbows to bring them closer to the ground. You should feel a stretch in your inner thighs and hips. Hold for 15-20 seconds, breathing deeply into the stretch.

3. Lunging Hip Flexor Stretch

Kneel on your right knee and place your left foot in front of you, creating a lunge position. Keep your torso upright and slowly lower your right knee towards the ground, feeling a stretch in the front of your right hip and thigh. Engage your core for stability and hold for 15-20 seconds. Repeat on the left side.

Quadriceps Stretches

1. Standing Quad Stretch

Stand tall with your feet hip-width apart. Bend your right knee and lift your right foot towards your glutes, using your right hand to hold onto your ankle. Keep your knees close together as you feel the stretch in the front of your right thigh. Hold for 15-20 seconds and then switch to the left leg.

2. Lying Quadricep Stretch

Lie face down on a mat or comfortable surface. Bend your right knee and bring your heel towards your glutes. Reach back with your right hand, grasping your right ankle. Gently pull your heel closer to your glutes while keeping your thighs parallel to each other. Hold this stretch for 15-20 seconds on each side.

3. Seated Quadricep Stretch

Sit on the ground with your legs stretched out in front of you. Bend your right leg and bring your right foot towards your glutes, placing it on the ground. Use your right hand to support your upper body as you gently lean back onto your right hand. Feel the stretch in your front right thigh. Hold for 15-20 seconds before alternating legs.

1. Standing Forward Fold

Stand tall with your feet hip-width apart. Slowly hinge at your hips, allowing your upper body to fold forward. Keep your knees slightly bent if needed. Reach for your shins, ankles, or the ground, depending on your flexibility. Feel the stretch in the back of your legs and hold for 15-20 seconds, focusing on relaxed breathing.

2. Seated Hamstring Stretch

Sit on the ground and extend your legs in front of you. Bend your left knee and place your left foot against the inside of your right thigh. Rotate your upper body towards your right leg and then slowly fold forward, reaching for your right ankle or foot. Feel the stretch in your right hamstring. Hold for 15-20 seconds before alternating legs.

3. Standing Hamstring Stretch

Stand tall with your feet hip-width apart. Take a step forward with your right foot and flex your right foot, toe pointing upwards. Slowly hinge at your hips, leaning forward, and reach towards your right foot with both hands. Keep your back straight and feel the stretch in the back of your right thigh. Hold for 15-20 seconds before alternating legs.

1. Wall Calf Stretch

Stand with your feet hip-width apart, facing a wall. Place your hands against the wall at shoulder height and step your right foot back. Keep your right foot flat on the ground and your right leg straight. Lean forward until you feel a stretch in your right calf. Hold for 15-20 seconds and then switch to the left leg.

2. Downward Dog

Begin by performing a push-up with your hands shoulder-width apart and your feet hip-width apart.

Lift your hips to the ceiling, keeping your legs as straight as possible. Press your heels towards the ground, feeling the stretch in your calves. Hold for 15-20 seconds as you relax into the pose, focusing on your breath.

3. Seated Calf Stretch

Sit on the ground and extend your legs in front of you. Place a towel or strap around the ball of your right foot and hold onto the ends with your hands. Pull the towel or strap towards you, flexing your right foot in the process. Feel the stretch in your right calf and hold for 15-20 seconds. Repeat on the left side.

By regularly incorporating these lower body stretches into your routine, you can improve flexibility, prevent muscle imbalances, and enhance your overall lower body mobility. Remember to perform these stretches gently and within your comfort zone. Enjoy the benefits of having limber and healthy lower body muscles.

Chapter 4: Core Stretches

Welcome to this chapter, where we will focus on stretching your core muscles. Your core is the foundation of your body and plays a vital role in maintaining stability, balance, and proper posture. By incorporating these core stretches into your routine, you can improve flexibility, reduce the risk of injuries, and enhance your overall core strength. This chapter is divided into three subchapters, targeting different areas of your core. Remember to warm up your body before attempting these stretches.

1. Seated Forward Bend

Sit on the ground and extend your legs in front of you. Take a deep breath in, lengthening your spine, and as you exhale, slowly hinge forward at the hips. Reach for your toes or shins while keeping your back flat. Feel the stretch in your abdominal muscles and hold for 15-20 seconds. Inhale as you gently return to your starting posture.

2. Standing Side Bend

Place your hands on your hips and stand with your feet hip-width apart. Inhale deeply, lengthening your spine, and as you exhale, slowly lean to the right side while sliding your right hand down your thigh. Feel the stretch along the left side of your body, focusing on your left oblique muscles. Hold for 15-20 seconds before alternating sides.

3. Supine Twist

Lie flat on your back with your arms extended to the sides, forming a T shape. Bring your knees to your chest by bending them. Exhale as you gently drop both knees to the right side, keeping your shoulders on the ground. Feel the stretch across your abdominal muscles and hold for 15-20 seconds.

Inhale as you bring your knees back to the center and repeat on the left side.

Lower Back Stretches

1. Child's Pose

Start on your hands and knees, then slowly sit back onto your heels. Extend your arms forward and lower your forehead to the ground, relaxing your entire body. Feel the stretch in your lower back as you breathe deeply for 15-20 seconds. Allow your spine to lengthen and your hips to sink towards your heels, creating a gentle traction effect on your lower back.

2. Cat-Cow Stretch

Begin on your hands and knees, positioning your wrists beneath your shoulders and your knees beneath your hips. As you inhale, arch your back, drawing your belly towards the floor and lifting your gaze upwards (cow position). Exhale as you round your spine towards the ceiling, tucking your chin towards your chest (cat position). Repeat this flowing movement for 5-10 breaths, gradually increasing the range of motion.

3. Standing Forward Fold with Hand Clasp

Stand with your feet hip-width apart and your fingers interlaced behind your back. On an exhale, slowly hinge forward at the hips, allowing your arms to come overhead and your hands to reach towards the ground. Feel the stretch in your lower back and shoulders. Hold for 15-20 seconds, breathing deeply into the stretch. Inhale as you slowly come back up to a standing position, releasing your hands.

Oblique Stretches

1. Seated Oblique Stretch

Sit on the ground and extend your legs in front of you. Cross your right leg over your left leg, placing your foot flat on the ground. Inhale deeply, lengthen your spine, and as you exhale, twist your torso to the right, placing your right hand behind you for support. Gently press your left elbow against your right knee, deepening the stretch in your oblique muscles. Hold for 15-20 seconds before alternating sides.

2. Standing Side Reach

Stand with your feet hip-width apart and raise your right arm overhead, bending it slightly. Inhale deeply, lengthening your spine, and as you exhale, lean to the left side, feeling the stretch along your right side body. Imagine reaching towards the ceiling with your right fingertips. Hold for 15-20 seconds before alternating sides.

3. Seated Russian Twist

Sit on the ground, knees bent and feet flat on the floor. Lean back slightly, keeping your back straight. Interlace your fingers and extend your arms straight out in front of you. Inhale deeply, and as you exhale, twist your torso to the right, rotating your arms and shoulders with you. Hold for 15-20 seconds and then twist to the left side.

By incorporating these core stretches into your routine, you will unlock the potential for improved stability, flexibility, and overall core strength.

Chapter 5: Full Body Stretches

Welcome to this chapter, where we will dive into the world of full-body stretches. Within this chapter, we will explore various stretching techniques that target different areas of your body. These stretches are not only beneficial for enhancing flexibility, but they also help in improving blood circulation and increasing your overall range of motion. By incorporating these stretches into your routine, you can experience a deeper sense of relaxation and enhance your physical performance.

1. Shoulder Stretch

Stand tall, feet hip-width apart. Extend your left arm out straight in front of you at shoulder height. Take your right arm and gently hook it under your left arm, just above the elbow. Slowly pull your left arm towards your chest until you feel a comfortable stretch in your shoulder. Hold for 15-20 seconds before alternating sides.

2. Pec Stretch

Stand beside a door frame or wall corner. Extend your left arm out to the side and place your forearm against the door frame, creating a 90-degree angle with your arm. Take a step forward with your left foot, allowing your body to lean forward slightly. You should feel a gentle stretch across your chest and front shoulder. Hold for 15-20 seconds before alternating sides.

3. Upper Trapezius Stretch

Sit or stand with your spine tall. Tilt your head gently to the right, bringing your right ear to your right shoulder. Place your right hand over your left temple and apply a gentle downward pressure to deepen the stretch. You should feel a release in the left side of your neck and shoulder. Hold for 15-20 seconds before alternating sides.

1. Hip Flexor Lunge

Start in a lunge position with your right foot forward, your knee bent at a 90-degree angle, and your left knee resting on the ground. Lace your hands on your right thigh and hold for support. Gently shift your weight forward, feeling a deep stretch in the front of your left hip. Hold for 15-20 seconds before alternating sides

2. Calf Stretch

Stand facing a wall or sturdy support. Keep your left foot forward, ensuring your knee is slightly bent, while your right leg extends straight behind you. Place your hands on the wall and lean forward, keeping both heels on the ground. You should feel a light stretch in your right calf region. Hold for 15-20 seconds before alternating sides

Remember to listen to your body, breathe deeply, and never force a stretch beyond your comfort level. By incorporating these full-body stretches into your routine, you can improve your flexibility, increase blood circulation, and promote a greater sense of relaxation and well-being. Enjoy the journey to a more flexible and revitalized body!

Chapter 6: Specific Stretching Exercises for Back Pain Relief

Welcome to this chapter, where we will focus on specific stretching exercises that target the back to provide relief from back pain. Back pain is a common issue that affects many individuals, and incorporating these stretches into your routine can help alleviate discomfort, improve mobility, and strengthen the muscles supporting your spine. In this chapter, we will explore solutions for the upper back and the lower back with detailed stretches that you can follow to alleviate back pain and promote a healthier back.

1. Shoulder Blades Squeeze

Stand or sit with your back straight. Start by bringing your shoulder blades together, squeezing them tightly as if you're trying to hold a pencil between them. Hold this position for 10-15 seconds, feeling the stretch across your upper back. Release and repeat for 2-3 repetitions.

2. Doorway Stretch

Stand facing a doorway with your arms extended to the sides at shoulder height. Bend your elbows and place your forearms on the doorframe, creating a 90-degree angle with your arms. Slowly lean forward, allowing your chest to move through the doorway while keeping your arms in position. You should feel a gentle stretch in the front of your shoulders and chest. Hold this position for 20-30 seconds and repeat for 2-3 repetitions.

3. Thread the Needle Stretch

Start on all fours, with your hands directly under your shoulders and knees under your hips. Extend your right arm out to the side, reaching towards the ceiling. Without moving your hips, thread your right arm under your left arm, resting your right shoulder and cheek on the mat. Hold for 20-30 seconds after relaxing into the stretch. Return to the

starting position slowly and repeat on the other side.
Complete 2-3 repetitions per side.

Lower Back Stretches

1. Glute Stretch

Lie flat on your back with your legs extended. Bend your right knee and cross it over your left thigh, bringing your right ankle to rest on your left thigh. Slowly pull your left knee towards your chest, feeling a stretch in your right glute. Hold for 20-30 seconds before switching sides. Repeat 2-3 times per side.

2. Sphinx Pose

Lie on your stomach with your forearms on the ground, elbows directly beneath your shoulders. Press through your forearms and lift your head, chest, and upper abdomen off the mat, keeping your pelvis grounded. A mild stretch should be felt in your lower back. Hold this position for 20-30 seconds, focusing on steady breathing. Release back down and repeat for 2-3 repetitions.

3. Lying Knee Twist

Lie flat on your back with your legs extended. Bring your knees to your chest by bending them. Drop your knees to the right slowly, keeping your upper back and shoulders firmly planted on the mat. You can use your left hand to gently guide your knees deeper into the stretch. Hold for 20-30 seconds, then switch sides. Repeat 2-3 times per side.

Incorporating these specific stretching exercises for back pain relief into your routine can help alleviate discomfort, improve flexibility, and strengthen the muscles supporting your back. Remember to listen to your body, focus on proper form, and never push yourself beyond your comfort level. Take care of your back and enjoy the benefits of a stronger and more flexible spine!

Bonus Chapter: 5 Minute Stretching Routines for Different Times of the Day

In this chapter, we will explore the importance of stretching and how it can benefit your upper body. Stretching is a crucial aspect of any fitness routine as it helps improve flexibility, muscle mobility, and prevents injuries. This chapter focuses specifically on stretching routines for different times of the day, allowing you to incorporate stretching into your daily routine. Whether you need to energize in the morning, relieve tension during breaks, or wind down in the evening, we have routines tailored to meet your needs.

Morning Energizers

Start your day off right by incorporating these stretching routines into your morning routine. These exercises will help awaken your muscles, improve blood flow, and prepare you for the day ahead.

Routine 1: Dynamic Upper Body Stretching

- **Arm Circles:**

Stand with feet shoulder-width apart. Extend your arms out to the sides and make circular motions with your arms. Gradually increase the size of the circles, alternating between clockwise and counterclockwise directions for 30 seconds.

- **Neck Stretches:**

Stand tall and slowly tilt your head to the left, bringing your left ear towards your shoulder. Hold for 10-15 seconds and then repeat on the right side. Repeat this stretch twice or three times on each side.

Routine 2: Standing Shoulder Opening

- **Shoulder Rolls:**

Stand with feet shoulder-width apart. Roll your shoulders in a circular motion, starting with small circles and gradually increasing the size. Roll forward for 10 repetitions and then backward for 10 repetitions.

- **Chest Stretch**

Stand with feet hip-width apart and clasp your hands behind your back. Stretch and straighten your arms away from your body, until you start feeling a stretch in your chest. Hold for 15-20 seconds and release.

Midday Tension Relief

Take a break from your busy day and relieve tension in your upper body with these stretching routines.

These exercises can be done anywhere, even in your office or during a short break, to promote relaxation and reduce stiffness.

Routine 1: Seated Upper Body Stretching

- **Shoulder Shrugs:**

Sit tall in your chair and raise your shoulders towards your ears, feeling the tension build. Hold for a few seconds and then release, allowing your shoulders to drop down. Repeat this exercise for 10 repetitions.

- **Wrist and Hand Stretches:**

Extend your right arm straight in front of you, palm facing up. Use your left hand to gently pull back your fingers, feeling a stretch in your forearm. Hold for 15 seconds and then repeat on the other side.

Routine 2: Neck and Upper Back Release

- **Neck Rolls:**

Sit upright with your feet flat on the ground. Slowly rotate your head in a circular motion, bringing your chin towards your chest, then to the left shoulder, back, and to the right shoulder. Complete 5 rotations in one direction and then switch to the other direction.

- **Upper Back Stretch:**

Interlace your fingers in front of you and push your palms away from your body. Round your upper back, pressing your palms forward and feeling a stretch between your shoulder blades. Hold for 15-20 seconds and release.

Wind down at the end of the day and promote relaxation with these stretching routines. These exercises will help release tension, reduce muscle soreness, and prepare your body for a restful night's sleep.

Routine 1: Supine Upper Body Stretching

- **Spinal Twist:**

Lie on your back, legs bent, feet flat on the ground. Extend your arms out to the sides in a T position. Slowly lower both knees to the right side, keeping your shoulders flat on the ground. Hold for 15 seconds alternate and repeat on the opposite side.

- **Child's Pose:**

Kneel on the floor and then sit back on your heels softly. Extend your arms forward and lower your chest towards the ground, allowing your forehead to rest on the mat. Hold this position for 30 seconds, focusing on deep breathing.

Routine 2: Wall Upper Body Stretching

- **Wall Angels:**

Stand with your back against a wall and press your entire spine against it. Bend your elbows at a 90-degree angle and, keeping them pressed against the wall, slide your arms up and then down as far as you comfortably can. Repeat this motion for 10-15 repetitions.

- **Overhead Arm Clasps:**

Stand with your feet shoulder-width apart and extend your arms straight overhead. Clasp your hands together, palms facing upward, and push your arms slightly backward to feel a stretch in your upper back and shoulders. Hold for 20 seconds and release.

Remember, when it comes to stretching, you have to be consistent. Whether you choose to incorporate these routines in the morning, during the day, or in the evening, make it a habit to prioritize stretching for a healthier and more flexible upper body.

Chapter 7: Stretching for Improved Flexibility and Mobility

In this chapter, we will dive into the realm of stretching for improved flexibility and mobility. Flexibility is essential for maintaining a wide range of motion in your joints, while mobility refers to the ability to move freely and efficiently. By incorporating stretching routines specifically designed to enhance flexibility and mobility, you can increase your overall physical performance and reduce the risk of injuries. In this chapter, we will explore effective stretching routines that target various muscle groups to help you achieve optimal flexibility and mobility.

Flexibility Boosters

Here, we will focus on stretching routines that promote flexibility, allowing your muscles to lengthen and increase joint range of motion.

Routine 1: Hamstring Stretch

Place your feet hip-width apart. Bend forward at the hips slowly, maintaining your back straight. Reach your hands towards the ground, allowing them to hang naturally or resting them on your shins. Hold this position for 20-30 seconds, feeling the stretch in your hamstrings.

Routine 2: Hip Flexor Stretch

Stand with your feet placed together. Take a large step forward with your right foot, bending your knee at a 90-degree angle. Keep your left leg straight behind you. Lower your hips until you feel a stretch at the front of your left hip. Maintain this position for 20-30 seconds on both sides.

Mobility Enhancers

Here, we will explore stretching routines that specifically target improving mobility. These exercises aim to increase the range of motion in your joints, allowing for better flexibility and movement patterns.

Routine 1: Shoulder Mobility

Stand with your feet shoulder-width apart. Extend your arms out to the sides and make circular motions with your arms. Gradually increase the size of the circles, alternating between clockwise and counterclockwise directions for 30 seconds.

Routine 2: Spine Mobility

Start on all fours, aligning your wrists under your shoulders and your knees under your hips. Inhale and arch your back, lifting your chest upward, and tilting your pelvis downward (cow pose). Exhale and round your back, dropping your head and tucking your tailbone under (cat pose). Repeat this flow for 8-10 repetitions.

Full Body Flexibility and Mobility

In this subchapter, we will combine flexibility and mobility exercises to create a comprehensive full-body stretching routine. These exercises will target multiple muscle groups, enhancing overall flexibility and mobility.

Routine 1: Sun Salutations

- Mountain Pose: Stand tall, feet together, and arms at your sides.

- Forward Fold: Exhale and hinge at the hips, folding forward and bringing your hands towards the ground.

- Lunge: Inhale and step your right foot back into a lunge position, keeping your left knee stacked over your left ankle.

- Downward Dog: Exhale and push back into a downward dog pose, pressing your palms and heels into the ground.

- Plank Pose: Inhale and shift forward into a high plank position, creating a straight line from your head to your heels.

- Repeat the sequence on the opposite side, starting with the lunge.

Routine 2: Spinal Twist and Hip Opener

- Seated Twist: Sit on the ground and extend your legs in front of you. Place your right foot outside your left thigh by bending your right knee. Inhale and lengthen your spine, then exhale and twist towards the right, placing your left elbow on the outside of your right knee for leverage. Maintain the hold for 20 seconds and alternate to the other side.

- Butterfly Stretch: Sit on the ground and bring the soles of your feet together, allowing your knees to fall out to the sides. Gently press your knees towards the ground while lengthening your spine, feeling a stretch in your hips. Hold for 20-30 seconds.

By incorporating these stretching routines into your fitness regimen, you can gradually improve your flexibility and mobility. Enjoy the benefits of increased flexibility and mobility in your everyday movements and activities.

Chapter 8: Incorporating Stretching into Daily Life

In this chapter, we will explore the art of incorporating stretching into your daily life. Stretching shouldn't be limited to just workout sessions or specific times of the day. It is a practice that can be seamlessly integrated into your daily routine, improving your overall flexibility, mobility, and overall well-being. In this chapter, we will discuss various ways you can easily and effectively include stretching in your day-to-day activities, ensuring that you reap the benefits of increased flexibility throughout your entire day.

Stretching at Home

Home stretches can be done in the morning to wake up your body, during breaks or downtime throughout the day, or in the evening to unwind and relax.

Waking Up with Morning Stretches

Start your day by taking a few minutes to stretch your whole body. Simple movements like reaching your arms overhead, twisting your torso gently, or doing a gentle forward fold can help your muscles wake up and prepare for the day ahead.

Stretch Breaks Throughout the Day

Incorporate short stretching breaks into your day whenever you have some downtime. Take a break from sitting or standing in the same position for extended periods by doing a quick stretch routine. Stretch your arms, legs, and neck to release tension and improve blood circulation.

Stretching at Work

Here, we will explore how you can integrate stretching into your work routine, even if you have a desk job. These stretches will help counteract the negative effects of prolonged sitting and promote better posture and overall well-being in the workplace.

Desk Stretches

Incorporate stretching exercises that can be done discreetly at your desk. Try neck stretches, shoulder rolls, wrist and forearm stretches, and seated twists to alleviate tension and improve circulation during work breaks.

Active Breaks

Take short active breaks throughout the day by walking around the office, climbing stairs, or doing simple standing stretches like calf raises, lunges, or reaching for the sky to energize your body and promote mobility.

Stretching in Everyday Activities

Here, we will discuss how you can incorporate stretching into your everyday activities, making it a seamless part of your routine and helping to improve your flexibility without disrupting your schedule.

Stretching while Waiting

Utilize waiting time during daily activities by incorporating stretches. Whether standing in line at the grocery store, waiting for a bus, or waiting for the coffee machine, perform simple stretches like calf raises, toe touches, or side stretches to make efficient use of this downtime.

Stretching during Chores

Turn everyday household chores into stretching opportunities. For example, while folding laundry, perform lunges or squats in between folds. While vacuuming, engage in calf raises or gentle twisting motions to activate different muscle groups.

Chapter 9: Tips for Long-Term Success and Results

In this chapter, we will be discussing tips and strategies for achieving long-term success and sustainable results. By now, you have learned various techniques and methods to help you reach your goals, but it is equally important to maintain those achievements in the long run.

As you continue reading, I will address the common challenges that arise when striving for long-term success and provide you with practical tips to overcome them. We will explore strategies to sustain motivation, develop consistency, and leverage your achievements to propel you forward. By implementing these tips, you will be equipped with the necessary tools to ensure lasting success and continue progressing on your journey.

Now, let's dive into the chapter and discover how you can set yourself up for long-term success and experience transformative results.

- **Set Clear and Realistic Goals:**

One of the keys to long-term success is to establish clear and achievable goals. Take the time to define what you want to accomplish and break it down into smaller, manageable steps. By setting realistic and concrete goals, you can stay focused and maintain the motivation needed to succeed over the long term.

- **Develop Consistency:**

Consistency is crucial when it comes to long-term success. Create a consistent routine that includes regular actions towards your goals. Whether it's dedicating a specific time each day to work on your projects or maintaining healthy habits, consistency breeds progress. It may be challenging at times, but developing discipline and committing to your goals will yield significant results in the long run.

- **Embrace Continuous Learning:**

Successful individuals never stop learning and growing. To achieve sustainable results, it's important to embrace a mindset of continuous learning. Seek out new knowledge, skills, and techniques relevant to your field. Stay up-to-date with industry trends and innovations. By expanding your knowledge base, you can adapt to changes and remain at the forefront of your industry.

- **Surround Yourself with Supportive People:**

Building a network of like-minded individuals who support your goals is crucial for long-term success. Surround yourself with individuals that motivate and inspire you to improve. Seek mentors who can provide guidance and accountability. By fostering positive relationships, you create a support system that can bolster your achievements and provide invaluable advice during challenging times.

- **Practice Self-Care and Manage Stress:**

Taking care of your physical and mental well-being is essential for maintaining long-term success.

Make time for self-care activities, such as exercise, meditation, and hobbies that rejuvenate your mind and body. Additionally, learn effective stress management techniques to prevent burnout and stay motivated. Remember, your well-being is the foundation on which your success is built.

- **Celebrate Milestones and Reflect on Achievements:**

Celebrating milestones along your journey helps to reinforce feelings of accomplishment and motivation. Take the time to acknowledge and reward yourself when you reach significant milestones. Consider your accomplishments and how far you've come. This not only boosts your confidence but also provides the motivation to keep pushing forward towards your long-term goals.

- **Adapt and Evolve:**

Flexibility and adaptability are key traits for long-term success Accept change and be willing to alter your strategies as needed. Evaluate your progress regularly and make necessary adjustments to your goals and action plans. By staying open-minded and adaptable, you can navigate through any roadblocks and challenges that may arise, ensuring your long-term success.

Remember, success is not an overnight phenomenon. It's a journey that requires perseverance, commitment, and continuous improvement. By incorporating these tips into your life, you will enhance your chances of long-term success and reap the rewards of your hard work. Stay focused, stay motivated, and never underestimate your potential to achieve great things in the long run.

Chapter 10: Conclusion and Final Thoughts

Dear friend,

As we near the end of this book, I want to take a moment to connect with you on a personal level. I understand that your journey towards success is not an easy one. The challenges, doubts, and uncertainties you face can be overwhelming at times. But remember, you are not alone. We have walked this path together, unraveling the secrets to long-term success.

Throughout these pages, I have shared with you the strategies, insights, and wisdom I have gathered over the years. My hope is that you have found the answers to your burning questions, and that this book has ignited a flame of inspiration within you.

In this journey, it is essential to be patient and kind to yourself. Acknowledge the progress you have made thus far, no matter how insignificant it may seem.

As we conclude our journey together, I want you to continue practicing self-care and prioritizing your well-being. You are the most significant asset on this path to success, and taking care of yourself is crucial. Nurture your physical, mental, and emotional health.

In closing, I want to express my gratitude for allowing me to be a part of your journey towards long-term success. I am humbled and honored to have shared this knowledge with you. My ultimate wish is that this book has provided you with the guidance, motivation, and inspiration needed to unlock your fullest potential.

Embrace your dreams, believe in yourself, and never cease your pursuit of greatness. You have what it takes to achieve long-term success.

Wishing you nothing but the best as you begin on this journey,

Nathan Anderson.

Thank you for purchasing and reading this book. I sincerely hope that you have found the solution to your problem in the pages of this book. If you have enjoyed reading this book, please leave a kind review so others can find the book and also get the help they need.